Candida

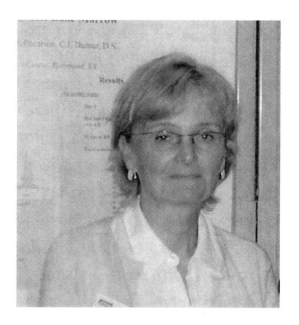

CANDIDA
AND
PARKINSON'S DISEASE

Candida and Parkinson's Disease

Is there a connection between your former husband's PD and the health problems you were experiencing?

LIDIA EPP: Yes, I think I need to start from the beginning. We were married in 1990 and it was probably about a year later I started to experience some issues with my health that I hadn't experienced ever before. There was of course at that point absolutely no connection to anything – I just started to notice strange new things about my health popping up here and there. Let me tell you a little about those health issues as it later became obvious they're part of a larger story.

About a year into our marriage I developed some skin issues and went to see a dermatologist. He told me that these were just age spots, which was kind of strange because I was 30. He also said it could be connected to me taking oral contraceptives and I shouldn't worry too much about it, a lot of women have

Candida and Parkinson's Disease

similar problems and it's nothing of concern. I also noticed kind of irregular freckle-like spots on my skin. Another strange thing that happened to me around the same time as that I stopped tanning. I used to tan easily and I spent a lot of time outdoors. I noticed I wasn't tanning anymore no matter how many hours I spent outside playing tennis or walking or working in a garden. I just didn't tan. I also noticed dark blotches on my skin. Those were my first symptoms.

About a year later I developed several so-called seasonal allergies. Symptoms ranged from stuffy nose, sneezing and watery eyes to really debilitating severe headaches; especially in the spring during the pollen season. I never had any problems with allergies and suddenly I was taking different nasal sprays and allergy medications – Claritin or whatever was available at the time and it really didn't alleviate my problem. I was told by my family physician that I have to resign

Candida and Parkinson's Disease

to the fact that sometimes later in life we can develop seasonal allergies and there's nothing that unusual about it. So I took my Nasonex and Claritin and walked around with watery eyes and sneezing 20 times at a time, thinking that's just the way life's going to be for me.

Other symptoms crept up one at a time as well. I noticed my back was hurting more often. I never had problems with my back before and suddenly I was experiencing severe pains in my lower and mid-back. I went to see the chiropractor and was told that I developed some mild to moderate spurs in my vertebrae. The chiropractor helped me some but not that much. I had to suffer through bouts of pain that would go away, but then would come back again. There were several of those symptoms that were seemingly unrelated to one another.

Around '96 - '97 my x-husband noticed some very disturbing symptoms in himself

Candida and Parkinson's Disease

and eventually – long story short – he went to see our family physician who sent him immediately to see a neurologist. He was diagnosed with an early onset of Parkinson's disease. He was 43 at the time. Back then of course we didn't see any connection between my seasonal allergies, back pain, migraines and my x-husband's diagnosis of Parkinson's disease. We didn't know that they all had a common denominator.

We led a very active lifestyle; we were both avid tennis players and runners. My husband tried to continue with those activities but it was increasingly difficult. His Parkinson's was progressing rapidly. His PD was not very responsive to the initial treatment. I don't recall the original therapy, but I'm certain that part of it was levodopa. It took quite some time and large doses of medication to see any improvement. Few months after the diagnosis my x-husband got in touch with a renowned neuropathologist from a very

Candida and Parkinson's Disease

prestigious medical school and we were delighted to finally have a national authority on the subject to see him; things looked really promising. That was the doctor which first prescribed him Mirapex. There is much more awareness about Mirapex now, but back then it was still an experimental drug and he was enrolled as part of a clinical trial. There was absolutely nothing known about the side-effects of the Mirapex. My x-husband didn't respond to the treatment like his doctor had hoped for. Actually all of his Parkinson's meds helped him only to certain, rather small degree. The disease was progressing quite rapidly no matter what the dosage of the medication was. Symptoms were very pronounced and getting worse regardless of the levadopa and Mirpaex dosage. The doctor was quite disappointed and prescribed increasingly larger doses of Mirapex. As I'm sure some of you are aware of it now - and if not, perhaps you should - Mirapex has some

Candida and Parkinson's Disease

severe side-effects. They are mostly neuropsychiatric in nature. Obsessive-compulsive disorder kicks in, irrational, paranoid behavior, aggression; now there's a wealth of information about it online.

Unfortunately for me and my x-husband, as a result of his Mirapex therapy - he had all of the side-effects present and our life took a turn for worse. His personality changed drastically and soon our marriage was on the rocks. I sought help from medical professionals, psychologists, psychiatrists, neurologists. I contacted the neurologist that prescribed the Mirapex but he simply brushed me off. He was not aware of any side-effects, his advice to me was: "Just enjoy the life that you have. Maybe your husband's personality changed somewhat. Wouldn't your personality change if you had been diagnosed with Parkinson's?" I suppose there's a grain of truth to it, so I said, "Okay, I'll take the good with the bad."

Candida and Parkinson's Disease

Things however got progressively worse to the point where my x-husband decided that he wants out of marriage. His uncontrollable obsessive-compulsive symptoms literally took over his personality. At this time he was on heavy doses of Mirapex and levodopa but his Parkinson's was still progressing rapidly.

I moved out to another state and lost touch with him. In the meantime, from common friends I've heard stories that his Parkinson's is still progressing. My ex husband is a geneticist and due to the severity of his PD symptoms it became impossible to continue his career.

Eventually I met my current husband - Bob and a few years later we got married. We would have lived happily ever after, however - after about a year of marriage, Bob noticed that he suddenly became allergic to pollen; developed back pain, severe migraines and severe skin rashes. This is when I said to myself: This is not a

Candida and Parkinson's Disease

coincidence, it just cannot be. Actually, I have to praise Bob, who by profession is a pilot: he spent days and nights relentlessly researching, mostly on the internet, what possibly could be a mildly contagious disease that would cause those symptoms and take years to develop? It was three o'clock in the morning one day when he woke me up and said: "I've found it!" At this point we knew it's not a coincidence that we both - previously very healthy, middle-aged people - suddenly develop the same health issues. It happened to me when I married my x-husband, now Bob is married to me and a year later he developed the same symptoms.

What symptoms were you experiencing when you figured out the cause?

LIDIA EPP: Let me just tell you, I was a mess. If you find a list of chronic candidiasis symptoms and it's a long list - I would say I had 80% of them. I was fatigued, depressed, I had severe skin rashes, I had constant GI problems, and I

Candida and Parkinson's Disease

had severe migraines. My migraines were absolutely debilitating at this point, the kind of migraine that makes you nauseous and light sensitive. Two years earlier I had back surgery, I had herniated and eventually ruptured lower back disc. Candida does weaken your cartilage.

Bob's first symptoms, especially one that bothered him the most were skin rashes. He had severe skin problems after less than a year after we met. So it became more and more obvious that there is a common denominator to all of that and finally Bob made the connection. He told me: "Look, these are all those scientific publications, it's really not my piece of pie. Why don't you read it? I think that's the thing that we both have". That's when I started to dig into it and sure enough, the more I read the more it became obvious to me - we are dealing with chronic polysystemic candidiasis.

I have to say there's a lot of bad

Candida and Parkinson's Disease

information online. There's some very good information and then there is some really bad. Just because somebody posted it online doesn't make it so and people do post the strangest things. If you come unprepared and start reading indiscriminately, you can wind up with some strange websites and strange advice; that's just my word of caution to all who is going to do any research online on that issue.

My first question was - how do we get rid of it? That led me to Dr. Orion Truss, a physician – I don't know if he's around anymore[1] – he was a gentleman in his 80s when I met him in 2005. I just called and I asked if I can come to Birmingham, Alabama to be his patient. I was desperate and so was my husband. Orion

---

[1] Dr. Truss died in September 2009 at 86. He and his late wife, Susan Heaslett Truss, were married for fifty-six years and had five children. He was the proud grandfather of fourteen grandchildren and a growing number of great-grandchildren.

Candida and Parkinson's Disease

Truss, MD is the ultimate authority on the subject so I simply asked if there was any chance he could see us. To my delight, Dr. Truss said yes. Next thing I know, I was on a plane to Birmingham Alabama to see Dr. Truss. His practice was dedicated exclusively to treating patients with chronic candidiasis. It was such a relief to see him, he was the first person I could talk to and he didn't tell me that I am a hypochondriac, there was nothing wrong with me and I should just take some over-the-counter Claritin and everything is going to be fine. I forgot to mention - just prior to becoming Dr Truss patient I was diagnosed with something called aspecific environmental asthma which basically meant - you have something that looks like asthma, but we don't know what it is and we don't know where it came from. I had a shortness of breath, this kind of a heavy feeling in my chest and a persistent, dry cough. I was prescribed some sort of inhaler that had

Candida and Parkinson's Disease

absolutely no effect on my condition.

I need to back up a little bit. Before I went to see Dr. Truss I tried my luck with our family physician. Bob and I made an appointment to see our family physician together. We told her the story; she looked at us as we're from another planet and told us "Well, there is no such a thing like chronic candidiasis." We insisted that never the less that's what we believe we have. She answered us, "When I was in medical school, they didn't teach us about chronic candidiasis, other than feminine candida infection or infant's yeast infection on the gums". She thought we are one of those strange people who believe that they read something online, suddenly decided they know medicine and consider themselves almost professionals. I think she decided that we're both hypochondriacs; we talked ourselves into being sick, to have some kind of mysterious disease that doesn't exist. Finally she concluded that maybe I have

Candida and Parkinson's Disease

some kind of bacterial infection and prescribed me broad-spectrum antibiotics. Most of the broad spectrum antibiotics have an anti-inflammatory component. Candida does cause a lot of inflammation in the upper respiratory tract and GI tract, so if you're taking antibiotic that has that component; it actually helps. I did therefore feel somewhat better, but as soon as I would finish the course of the antibiotics my condition actually worsened.

So you can experience some relief from symptoms because of anti-inflammatory components in those drugs, but it doesn't mean that the drug is the one that you should be taking. That's exactly what happened to me with one antibiotic after another and one inhaler after another, I was really going downhill very fast. My back problems were simply debilitating, my migraines were just horrible. I had two, three days of every week being completely incapacitated due to my

Candida and Parkinson's Disease

migraines. That's when I decided to see Dr. Truss and it was truly the beginning of the rest of my life for me. When I explained him my symptoms, how I was feeling, he would literally finish my sentences for me! It was such a relief. Finally I'm sitting at the doctor's office and here is a medical professional who knows what I'm talking about, who doesn't think I'm crazy and I'm just talking myself into being sick. He knows my symptoms and in the end, tells me that he's going to help me. That's how I started the Nystatin therapy. It's an anti-fungal medication. It's actually given to infants for oral thrush and it has no side-effects; if you take too much of it you might get nauseous, but that's all. Actually Nystatin is considered to be an antibiotic - Anti-biotic - one live organism that eradicates another organism, so this is bacteria that kills the fungi. It was discovered by a couple of microbiologists in 1950 on a dairy farm in New York State

Candida and Parkinson's Disease

- hence the name Nystatin. There was one farm in New York State that cows never had any fungal diseases, they took samples from that farm and discovered that the bacterium that is on cow's skin is what protects them from fungal infections. Nystatin is the purified powdered form of that bacterium and that's what it does; it feeds on yeast.

The powdered form is needed for the treatment of the chronic candidiasis as it is the most effective form. Most physicians prescribe it in a solution that contains a lot of sugar and that is the last thing you want when you have a Candida infection. I didn't know it back then, but Dr. Truss told me the only form of Nystatin that would work was that pure powdered form. You just mix it up with a little bit of water and drink it three times a day. It tastes horrible, but - it works!

How can you get Nystatin?

LIDIA EPP: I bought it at the

Candida and Parkinson's Disease

compounding pharmacy in Birmingham, Alabama. It has to have a prescription and the best chance of getting on Nystatin therapy is to see a homeopathic doctor. Now - here is a word of caution - Nystatin is a very important segment of that therapy, but it's not the whole thing. So please don't get an impression that if you just find somebody who can prescribe Nystatin - you will get well. It is only a portion of the story.

Dr Truss wrote a book, it's called Missing Diagnosis. This is the best book that I've seen on the subject of chronic Candida. Dr. Truss is extremely knowledgeable on the subject. He really researched the issue and he is actually the first one that named and diagnosed the symptoms of chronic candidiasis. He was a practicing physician in the hospital and noticed some patients that had symptoms which now are known as chronic polysystemic candidiasis. Back then they were just patients that wouldn't respond well to any

Candida and Parkinson's Disease

conventional therapies. They complained of recurring cold-like symptoms, fatigue, allergies, migraines, fungal skin infections, etc. Dr Truss was the first one to make the connection between that array of vague symptoms and the overgrowth of fungal organism in the tissues. Recently Missing Diagnosis II *was published, Dr Orion Truss is the author of that book as well. He also wrote a number of articles on the subject published in the '80s. The first one, I have it here with his autograph actually; Metabolic abnormalities in patients with chronic candidiasis: the acetaldehyde Hypothesis, published 1983.*

Long story short, I saw a dramatic improvement in myself and Bob recovered very quickly as well. We stopped the condition very early; we didn't leave the symptoms untreated for many years, therefore didn't have that much damage done to our bodies. We were still relatively young, in our early 40s and were able to

Candida and Parkinson's Disease

get our health back. We were absolutely religious about the regimen that had to be followed for a complete recovery.

After half a year, I was basically symptom-free. I had my life back, which was absolutely amazing. You don't know how bad you feel until you start feeling better again. Then you look back and realize how many things you gave up on doing, how limited your life became because of the debilitating condition that took over your life. Then I realized how significant it was and how significant was the improvement. I looked back at my life when it all started and said, well, okay, there is still that connection. My health deteriorated after I met my x-husband and then years later I passed this same health problem on to Bob. It has to be a mildly contagious condition that originated with my x-husband. Then I realized that he also had so many symptoms of chronic candidiasis. He had terrible problems with his GI. I think at some point he was

Candida and Parkinson's Disease

diagnosed with irritable bowel syndrome. He took large quantities of Zantac and Rolaids daily that did very little to alleviate his stomach upsets. He also had all these skin problems: fungal skin conditions and toe nail fungus. He would continuously try new anti-fungal treatments that did very little to help with those issues, fungal infections just kept coming back. I started to think about all those things and I said, "Well, okay. I'm quite certain that he had chronic candidiasis and I got it from him." Then I thought - is it possible that the Candida is the reason why he developed Parkinson's? Would that be part of the equation? He had no family history of Parkinson's and was in his early forties.

I started to look at it from that perspective and I did discover a connection which brings me right to the biochemical aspect of it.

Candida and Parkinson's Disease

What is the source of Candida? Can you get it from eating certain foods?

LIDIA EPP: Absolutely, yes. It is a 'live' yeast. The source of my problems with Candida was from contact with my x-husband, but you can develop the problem all on your own. Basically it's any combination of several factors. It could be for example - a long term use of broad-spectrum antibiotics. I have seen a lot of articles online talking about teenagers with acne who were treated them with tetracycline - low doses for an extended period of time to keep the acne at bay. That is apparently a perfect recipe for just wiping out your healthy gut flora and replacing it with Candida.

Now, don't get me wrong, Candida is present in a healthy person's GI tract. It is needed actually. We need Candida albicans as a part of our intestinal flora, so it's not that evil entity that invades us; it's just the balance or the percentage of how much of the Candida is a part of your

Candida and Parkinson's Disease

gut flora. If you have a broad-spectrum long term antibiotic administered for months at the time, that basically kills all the friendly bacteria. Antibiotics are fungi and they kill the bacteria; that's kind of the other side of the Nystatin story. What are left are the fungi that will not be killed off by antibiotics which are fungi as well. Candida then is basically filling out the vacuum principle. So if you take broad-spectrum antibiotic, that is really a huge predisposing factor.

Now I'm getting into some medical stuff and I just want to make sure that everyone understands that I'm not a medical professional. This is my story and this is my opinion, this is what I think but by no means I am giving any medical advice to anybody. I can give my advice with what I would do if I would be in that situation again, but these are just conclusions that I came to by dealing with the problems myself.

Candida and Parkinson's Disease

I believe that we are all part of nature and nature likes balance. If we don't have a balanced diet it will eventually cause bad things happening with our body, I really believe that. But I don't know which one comes first, the chicken or the egg: is it a Candida that causes you to crave certain foods and keep your diet off-balance, or you keep your diet off-balance so then Candida's more likely to grow? If you eat a lot refined carbohydrates, if you eat a lot of sugar, flour, simple carbohydrates; these are food for Candida to put it simply. It needs simple carbohydrates to reproduce and once Candida starts growing, it depletes your body of sugars. Then you crave them more and you really don't crave them for yourself but rather for the invading organism that depletes your body from a normal balance of those – because you do need some carbohydrates that should be part of your healthy diet. But if Candida utilizes all of that, metabolizes it itself then your body

Candida and Parkinson's Disease

craves that, and if your body craves you eat more and then you feed more Candida so Candida grows really quickly and there you have a vicious cycle. So, yes, diet is a very important component, but does it come as a result of your Candida problem or you develop Candida problem because of your diet–I am not sure.

> Do Candida hang out only in the GI tract or do they float all over the body?

LIDIA EPP: I believe it spreads throughout the body but don't tell that to any traditional medicine GI specialist because he will laugh. Candida infection starts in your GI and then it spreads throughout the various tissues. I had a Candida in my lungs. That's why I had a hard time breathing. During that time when I had really severe Candida infection I literally could hardly breathe; it was like somebody pushed on my chest and prevented me from breathing in. Ever since I became Candida-free I never experienced that again. It makes me believe that there was

Candida and Parkinson's Disease

a fungal overgrowth in my respiratory tract.

Can freckles and dark spots on the skin be evidence of Candida?

LIDIA EPP: I don't have any dark blotches on my skin anymore. Now interestingly enough, my x-husband always had those freckles but not so round and pronounced as regular freckles are. But these were basically darker blotches on the skin. For me, what was very characteristic when it comes to skin, it's that I stopped tanning. I think Candida utilizes pigment from your skin so you lose ability to tan. Being a person that spends a lot of time outdoors, I noticed that at the end of the summer, I was not tanned anymore, regardless of the amount of time I spent outdoors. If years back you did tan and now you cannot, it's another piece of evidence that you might have a Candida infection. The Candida invades your skin and prevents skin from the natural process of tanning which requires

Candida and Parkinson's Disease

pigment.

Another thing that is very important: if you're experiencing all of those various symptoms, the infection is severe. It's chronic, very serious fungal infection. Your body is trying to fight it off and that's why you would develop various allergies. The autoimmune system is just out of control. It doesn't know what to do with the invading fungal cells. Then you develop food allergies, chemical allergies, you can become allergic to smells. Women can become allergic to their perfumes.

Your immune system would say, "Okay, I'm on overload, I just don't know what to do so I'm going to react to everything or I'm not going to react to anything." That is so true when it comes to the fungal diseases. People that have Candida often develop other fungal diseases because the immune system just gives up on fungal antigens and say, "Okay, I guess these are

Candida and Parkinson's Disease

just parts of my skin; this is part of my body now so I have to allow them to exist." People with Candida infections will have toenail fungus, ringworm, tinea corporis; there are a lot of different fungal conditions that are opportunistic and are basically a result of your body's lack of defense against fungal organisms in general. I had a really bad case of ringworm that I promptly gave to my husband, it's highly contagious.

So there are a lot of those different components that come into play with the chronic candidiasis. And when you start to follow the trail, at some point it just all falls in place and it's like, "Oh wow, I have this and I have that, I didn't know it was all connected". Suddenly it's like a big puzzle that you look at and you now see a big picture, when before it was just separate little pieces that you would never put together as part of the same issue.

Candida and Parkinson's Disease

What else did you do to rid yourself of the over-abundance of Candida in your body?

LIDIA EPP: Again I would refer to the Missing Diagnosis, Dr. Truss' book. He spelled it out in detail. In general: you don't eat carbohydrates–you starve Candida because that's what Candida needs to metabolize in order to multiply and to live. Carbohydrates are the food that the organism will utilize in order to keep invading your tissues. So if you starve the organism by not ingesting anything that Candida can metabolize to support its life cycle, then you basically deprive it of its food source. And then, whatever is not killed off by the lack of food, you eliminate with the antifungal medication.

It is a very, very rigorous prescription but, believe me, I don't know how to stress it more; you cannot cheat. You cannot say, "Well, I'm just going to have this doughnut today and then I will go back on my diet tomorrow." I suppose it could

Candida and Parkinson's Disease

*work if you try just to lose some weight,
but if you are on an anti-Candida
regimen, you absolutely cannot do that.
It is like starting all over again. So it's
really a draconian diet, but it works. You
have to commit yourself 150%. You
cannot say, "Today I'm going to take it
easy on myself. I'm going to put some
sugar in my coffee". Or - "I really, really
like that pizza place, so I'm just going to
have one slice." You simply cannot do
that. To really follow this diet effectively
requires a great deal of commitment and
knowledge. I had to really sit down and
educate myself.*

*There are books that you can buy online
on nutritional food content, one of them
became sort of my Bible. It's a big book
with lists of all the food items and it has
the carbohydrates and calories content of
just about any food item you can think of.
You would need to focus on carbohydrates
of course. You have to stay on about 50 to
60 grams a day. It's nothing. It's one*

Candida and Parkinson's Disease

teaspoon of sugar, that's it. It's really hard and you would not believe where carbohydrates are hidden. Do you know how much sugar is in the spaghetti sauce? There are foods that you never think of that have high carbohydrate content.

You have to read every label of every food item and you have to walk around with a calculator and if by lunch you exceeded or are at your maximum for the day, then you just stick with salad. But even tomatoes have a lot of sugar. Carrots have a lot sugar; so not every vegetable will work. I have to tell you, it's a wonderful diet if you want to lose weight - I lost 20 pounds; actually I lost more than I wanted or that I should have. I was very skinny at the end of that diet. I stayed on that diet for two years. But you learn dos and don'ts, you learn what you can eat and what you cannot and it becomes easier.

The first few months it's terrible and also

Candida and Parkinson's Disease

you have the 'die-off' phenomenon where the Candida starts to die off and you feel terrible. You actually feel sick. You can even run fever – and I did for a few days – I felt like I had a flu, and it's probably not an appealing way to put it but basically when Candida starts dying off it gives out all different toxins and you feel sick because suddenly the living organism that used to invade your tissues is dying. For some people I heard it can take up to two weeks, for me it was three or four days; I felt terrible. If you do however stick with this diet through that period of time, after a few weeks suddenly there is a dramatic improvement. That was very encouraging to me because the diet is so draconian.

Can a person get rid of Candida in a few weeks?

LIDIA EPP: I hate to say it, but it is not a quick fix. You cannot do the Candida diet for a week and next Monday wake up and be healthy. There are no quick fixes. There is no easy, miracle pill that you take

Candida and Parkinson's Disease

and everything is good. You cannot expect to stick to the diet for a short period of time and then wake up in a couple of weeks feeling great. It requires a long haul commitment but it can be done.

I'm now enjoying my dark chocolate. I'm enjoying pizza occasionally. I'm not on a diet anymore at all. The whole experience did teach me how to eat wiser. When I go to the grocery store I still shop looking at the labels. I don't buy foods that are high in sugars and simple carbohydrates. I do eat much healthier as a result of it, but I think it's good and it really has nothing to do with Candida anymore but I just feel much better. If you stay on this Candida diet eventually you can go up on carbohydrates to 100 grams a day or so. After a few months you can ease your body back into some of that and if you feel relapse, if you start to feel sluggish, bloated, you start to feel symptoms of Candida again then you have to back up of course. But the first several months it's

Candida and Parkinson's Disease

very strict and there are no quick answers of how to get rid of it quickly.

LIDIA EPP: I contacted my x-husband and I told him about my findings; that I believe he has a Candida infection and I also believe that there is a connection between the Candida and the Parkinson's. My ex-husband is a geneticist. He listened to me carefully and then said: "You're right. You're absolutely right; I think you just figured out how to help me out with my Parkinson's." At that time he was not working professionally anymore, he was unable to do that. He had the deep brain stimulation (DBS) which didn't really work. DBS didn't give him the results that everybody was telling him that he would experience. He was having a really rough time with the Parkinson's which was really devastating him.

After our phone conversation - he went to

Candida and Parkinson's Disease

see Dr. Truss as well. I was told that it was astonishing; it was such a dramatic improvement. An old friend of mine who ran into him on the street one day told me that she could not believe her eyes; what a remarkable improvement it was. I don't know how he's doing now, but I understand a couple of years ago that he was still doing great. It's my understanding that he stayed on a very strict anti-Candida diet and after a while, he no longer needed the deep brain stimulation that didn't work well for him in the first place.

He told me a little story – and I hope he doesn't mind my sharing it with you now – he went to the University hospital where they did the deep brain stimulator implant. As I understand the procedure: you have a remote control switch which you can turn the stimulator in your brain on and off. They were doing some tests and asked him to turn it on first and then they would go through some mobility

Candida and Parkinson's Disease

tests with him to find out how he was doing. So they did the mobility test and said: "Oh, you are doing great. You see there is a significant improvement." Then he told them, "Well, I have a surprise for you. I didn't turn it on. It was off the entire time."

And they got mad at him. They said what did you do that for? It messes up our statistics. He asked: "Well, aren't you excited? I am much better, and I can tell you why I'm better. I found the reason. I know the cause of my Parkinson's and I'm curing it right now. Don't you want to know?" But they didn't even listen. They were so busy looking at the monitor, concerned how that's going to throw off all the statistics. They were not interested in his remarkable improvement, just worried the data is in the wrong column and how it's going to look. So my understanding is that he got much better and he was on his way to – I don't know whether it's a full recovery. It is my

Candida and Parkinson's Disease

opinion that he had it for so many years and there was so much damage done to his central nervous system, that he was not able to fully recover his motor ability and muscle functions. But it was my understanding the last time I talked to him, about four years ago, that he is doing remarkably better.

So, he got better, you got better and just to be clear, Bob, your current husband, is also now well?

LIDIA EPP: He was very early in the whole vicious cycle, so he recovered first actually. It took me a little longer to get to the point where I was back to normal but now my scar from my back surgery is the only permanent reminder of my past health problems. I don't have any allergies; I don't know what migraines are. We live out in the country and in the spring there is a lot of pollen in the air, but I don't have any allergies. I never take any Benadryl or Claritin. I spend a lot of

Candida and Parkinson's Disease

time outdoors and I do tan. I have no skin problems. Quite frankly, I'm a very healthy middle-aged person right now. I take no medicine of any kind and I am not on any diet. I know that carbohydrates are not a good thing to eat in excess, so I do watch what I eat in that respect. I don't like the sweet taste because I'm not used to sugar anymore and I prefer to keep it that way. So I'm doing great and Bob is fine and as far as I can tell, my x-husband is doing much better.

What is the connection between candidiasis and Parkinson's?

LIDIA EPP: The way Candida metabolizes carbohydrates is that it breaks it down to acetaldehyde, a compound that is directly involved in formation of salsolinol. Salsolinol is a neurotoxin that is selectively targeting dopamine receptors. So if you have millions of Candida cells in your body, they produce massive amounts of the acetaldehyde that travels through your blood to the brain where it's

Candida and Parkinson's Disease

transformed into the neurotoxin that targets your dopamine receptors. Salsolinol triggers apoptosis of dopaminergic neurons. Apoptosis is a fancy name for a programmed cell death.

Cells are kind of like little computers of sorts. They have several programs running simultaneously telling them to multiply, replicate, grow, whatever. They also have a program called apoptosis: when it's time to die, they engage that program which is a cascade of biochemical processes that tells a cell to die.

Salsolinol is a compound; it's a chemical that will trigger that apoptosis signal in dopaminergic neurons; it will not cause just any random cell to die. It specifically targets neurons that are associated with dopamine - dopamine receptors. So there is a vicious cycle and if you look at it, it's a very straight-forward chain reaction. There are reports and scientific papers

Candida and Parkinson's Disease

that discuss the elevated level of salsolinol in the spinal fluid of people with Parkinson's disease. Salsolinol also is present in urine of PD patients. So there is evidence to support this chain of causal events.

You wrote up your discovery and published it as a journal article?

LIDIA EPP: I started to look for papers connecting the source of increased salsolinol to Candida and the possibility of it triggering PD-like symptoms and to my astonishment, I didn't find any. Nobody wrote about it. I was just completely puzzled and thought maybe I'm missing something. Then I started to write emails to whoever wants to listen to me and that was mostly scientists that work in the field of pathology of Parkinson's. After knocking on a lot of different doors and talking to a lot of people who were very skeptical about my theory - I found myself pretty discouraged.

Candida and Parkinson's Disease

Finally I wrote to Dr. Boris Mravec in Slovakia; he is a distinguished professor of immunophysiology and endocrinology at the Bratislava Medical School. After so many failed attempts to interest scientists in my theory - I didn't really expect to hear from him. But on the very next day I got an email from the Dr. Mravec. I had to read it five times until it finally sank in –it read: "You have a groundbreaking theory. It is my assessment that you're theory's absolutely correct. Would you like to write a paper?" It really took me at least five times to read it to realize- oh my gosh, he believes me. That's how it all started and we emailed back and forth. I wrote an article, he made some additions and revisions and we got it published in his medical schools' journal in 2006. The article is titled Chronic Polysystemic Candidiasis as a Possible Contributor to Onset of Idiopathic Parkinson's Disease.

If somebody is interested out there in doing any research to prove (or disprove)

Candida and Parkinson's Disease

my theory - they can take it and run with it. This is not in the scope of my professional activities. I'm not a PD researcher and would never have any funds to conduct such a research. But I think it's a valid theory. Now I look back and I realize that it is one of the many connections of the whole process, the biochemical interaction between Candida metabolism, dopamine receptors pathology and the symptoms of Parkinson's; it is a very complex multileveled biochemical process.

I have some further thoughts on how this biochemical processes take place. There is a chemical called tissue transglutaminase. It's a very hot topic now in the field of pathology. There is a well researched, straight-forward connection between tissue transglutaminase and celiac disease. Candida is implicated in the onset of celiac disease and tissue transglutaminase is identified as the auto-antigen in celiac

Candida and Parkinson's Disease

disease. *Tissue transglutaminase catalyzes the formation of alpha-synuclein crosslinks in Parkinson's disease.*

Lewy bodies are alpha-synuclein aggregates in the brain of people with Parkinson's disease and are catalyzed by tissue transglutaminase, so there is another very straight-forward biochemical pathway that links: Candida with celiac disease, with symptoms of chronic candidiasis and with Parkinson's. I think the process if very complex and multifaceted, what I found out is just a little tip of an iceberg. The iceberg is still underwater, but it's all connected.

Transglutaminase or tTG is basically something that plays a role in Candida's life cycle?

LIDIA EPP: Yes. It stimulates the antibody formation against Candida. It triggers the immune response that results in inflammation in the gut in the presence of

Candida and Parkinson's Disease

Candida. Your body starts producing tissue transglutaminase and when tTG is produced in excess it in turn catalyzes the formation of the lewy bodies – the hallmark of Parkinson's disease in the brain. In the way - it causes dopamine receptors to die and form those aggregates in the substantia nigra. The Candida starts the cascade, part of it is the acetaldehyde formation, but also it induces your body to start producing tissue transglutaminase. By the way - tTG is also associated, there's a lot of publications on that subject, with the tissue injury. If you think about it - the lining of your intestine is injured by Candida albicans since it actually adheres to the intestine walls. So it starts a cascade of events and this is just another biochemical pathway of the same process, which is very complex and I'm sure I don't understand it fully. I don't think anybody understands it completely yet and there is no published research data linking all of

Candida and Parkinson's Disease

that together.

So it'd be nice to find some collaborators, some people who were willing to take this to the lab and do some rat studies and carry that further and do some case studies it sounds like?

LIDIA: This is really not my field, I'm a molecular biologist but I don't specialize in that field. This is totally out of my area of expertise. I can read a paper and understand it but this is not what I do for a living. I would love to hand it over to somebody who knows more on the subject of neuropathology of Parkinson's and who has the money and energy and interest in doing this. That would be fantastic. Regardless of how many husbands or ex-husbands are in my story, I truly believe that my theory has merit.

Is there a connection between a foot or toe fungus and Parkinson's symptoms?

LIDIA EPP: Yes, there could be a

Candida and Parkinson's Disease

connection. Chronic infection with Candida does lower immune response to other fungal conditions like skin conditions, so it probably is associated.

You see, if you suffer from chronic candidiasis you basically do not have a normal immune response to fungal diseases. Your body is pretty much defenseless against fungal pathogens. There are publications, that people with Candida and people with Parkinson's have problems with fungal diseases like skin conditions, toenail fungus, etc. I'm not saying that all the Parkinson's cases are induced by Candida, by no means.

I believe that Candida is a very possible component of that picture and that it produces neurotoxin. If on the top of it you have other predisposing factors, you will develop Parkinson's eventually. Parkinson's is a name for a set of symptoms and the causes of those symptoms can be different. It could be a

Candida and Parkinson's Disease

traumatic head injury, like Muhammad Ali; his story has to be completely unrelated to Candida.

My x-husband was a long-distance runner. He wanted to stay lean and not gain weight especially when he was training for a race. But he liked his tea really sweet and didn't want to put sugar in it so he used aspartame - NutraSweet in huge quantities. I believe that aspartame is a very potent neurotoxin; it is just the worst thing that you can put in your mouth. It is documented that it is selective neurotoxin. So there was another predisposing factor to his Parkinson's.

I believe that Candida infection is a huge predisposing factor to Parkinson's yet it might not be enough to trigger the onset of PD. Maybe you need another factor that will favor the development of PD; that will be the straw that breaks the camel's back. In my husband's case that was the aspartame, but it could be different things for different people. For instance, farmers that are exposed to pesticides in huge quantities – that could be a very large contributing factor. All our bodies are different; our weak points are in different places. PD is a very general description of symptoms that can be caused by any number of things.

How to Hear Lidia on Parkinsons Recovery Radio

Visit http://www.blogtalkradio.com/parkinsons-recovery and scroll back to find the show that aired March 23, 2011 featuring Lidia as my guest.

About Lidia Epp

Lidia M. Epp is a molecular biologist and lives in the Virginia countryside with her husband. For over twenty years she has been employed by several universities, where she has participated in research projects dealing with the molecular aspects of

Candida and Parkinson's Disease

disease detection and diagnosis. For ten of those twenty years she served as a research specialist in the clinical molecular diagnostics laboratory at the Medical College of Virginia. Currently, Lidia works at the Biology Department of the College of William and Mary, where she coordinates the activities of the departmental molecular core laboratory. In her spare time, she is an avid organic gardener. Lidia and her husband Bob enjoy spending time aboard their sailboat cruising the Chesapeake Bay. You can contact Lidia via her email: mailto:lidiaepp@gmail.com